the wheel
of the
woman

PRINTED IN THE UNITED STATES OF AMERICA

ISBN: 979-8-9883110-4-1

For information, address:
5 Two Press, LLC
PO box 535
Carson City, NV 89701

5twopress@gmail.com

Any and all content available in this book is made available solely for educational and informational purposes only, and does not constitute medical or other professional health care advice, diagnosis, or treatment. Always seek the advice of a qualified health professional or provider. Reliance on any information in this book is solely at your own risk. Neither the author or publisher can be held liable for any implied, punitive, special, incidental or other consequential damages arising directly or indirectly from any use of the content in this book, which is provided as is, and without warranties.

Cover Designed by: Kristen Rud
Names: Rud, Kristen, author
Title: The Wheel of the Woman: An Almanac for Women's Wellbeing.

the woman knows that stagnant waters will create stagnant beings.

therefore it is necessary to shift with the seasons; to sync with the moon; and to move with the sun to be at our truest nature.

table of contents

#wheelofthewoman

my magdalene lineage

◎ My Mother

Carole Walker (born 1968)

◎ My Grandmother

Joan Morton (7/22/1934 - 8/10/2002)

◎ My Great Grandmother

Emily Lefferts (9/9/1906 - 5/28/1989)

◎ My 2nd Great Grandmother

Anna Sacks (9/21/1877 - 7/01/1975)

◎ My 3rd Great Grandmother

Mary Benner (3/5/1849 - 2/16/1920)

◎ My 4th Great Grandmother

Hannah Fink (1812 - 2/12/1898)

◎ My 5th Great Grandmother

Maria Magdalena Miller (1/6/1780 - 10/2/1856)

◎ My 6th Great Grandmother

Mary Magdalene Bos (9/8/1744 - 9/28/1829)

◎ My 7th Great Grandmother

Maria Magdalena Streit Benner (1709-1770)

◎ My Grandmothers Beyond

My grandmother Joan was a short, round woman with a giant belly laugh that made her whole face turn red. She loved Frank Sinatra, Christmas, and had quite the gift for astrology and 'the mystics', if you will. She was the local astrologer and card reader for hundreds of people throughout her lifetime, even a few celebrities had her number memorized (that's like speed dial for the 70s and 80s, right?).

Just shy of ten years old, we pulled up to her house after a blazing drive across the summer desert. I ran in for a big, sweaty hug. That was my last hug from my favorite person. Grandma had a massive heart attack that day. She died a couple hours later. And a piece of me, that she was carefully cultivating, went dormant with her.

Fifth grade started a few weeks later, I rapidly put on weight and struggled socially. Doctors couldn't figure out what was 'wrong' with me, so over time they gave me the diagnosis of fibromyalgia. At 12 years old, I was marked with a less-than-understood autoimmune disorder, like a *Scarlet Letter*.

My Rite of Passage to Womanhood has begun. And the Wheel of the Woman is the map.

Xo, MM

I

what is
WOMAN?

in the beginning
what did they call her?
was the first woman really called
eve?

In English, we call her Woman, evolved from *wifman* "wife person" in Old English. The Scandinavians call her *Kvinne* or *Kvinna*, evolved from the Proto-Germanic word *Kwēniz*, meaning "wife" or "queen".

The etymology of Eve has its roots in the Latin name *Eva*. In turn, *Eva* originated from the Hebrew *Chavah* or *Havah*, which means "to breathe" and "to live" or "to give life". The traditional meaning of the name *Eve* is "life" or "living".

The Latin language still influences the name of Woman in modern French, Italian and Spanish languages. The French language refers to women as *Femme* derived from the Latin term *Femina*, which translates back to woman in English. The Italians call her *Donna*, with Latin roots that bring the translation to "lady" or "mistress of the house". The Spanish call her *Mujer*, also rebirthing from ancient Latin ancestors named *Mulier*. Some suspect that *Mulier* sprouted from the Latin term *Mollis* meaning "soft," while others believe it originated from *Mulgere*, which means "to breastfeed." ◎

Language is a living thing, constantly evolving and adapting to new circumstances. While the roots of a word may offer a glimpse into its original essence, they do not define its every aspect. Many words are imbued with multitudes of meanings, their essence shifting in the light of their surroundings.

It falls upon us, the inheritors of the title, to be open to the myriad of interpretations of Woman, and to be willing to deepen our understanding, as the tides of time ebb and flow. For it is through this graceful dance of interpretation and introspection that we can unravel the mysteries of Her, of Us, of You.

II

the birth of HER

"a rite of passage is

a series of rituals

designed to conduct an

individual from one social

state or status to another;

thereby affecting

transformations

both in society's

perceptions of the

individual and in the

individual's perception

of self."

-robbie davis floyd; phd

Her Story

Let's get technical for a second: A woman's eggs come with one X chromosome, while sperm can bring either an X or Y chromosome to the party. If sperm brings a Y, 'it's a boy!' But for the sake of this story, let's assume the sperm brings an X chromosome. Sperm meets egg. XX. Marked a girl; *determined by man*. Made to be a woman from the moment of conception. Designed to be placed inside the belly of the one who came before. As she emerges from her predecessor, she reveals a hidden beauty, a reminder that treasures often lie buried in the depths of the darkness, at the center. And we're sent off into this world, spending our whole lives trying to unravel the intricate layers of womanhood that have been placed upon us. Like a set of nesting dolls, intricately crafted and steeped in legend, traditions are passed down through feminine lineages. ◎

Maybe it's 'Eve's Curse' or maybe it's the greatest gift. Either way, we're marked from the beginning. Your Rite of Passage to Womanhood has begun.

The birth of Self initiates us into the world, and learning immediately begins through our senses. XX is now a girl, with a name and a human form. Hormones in her little body pique in the minutes immediately after birth, allowing her to be alert. The primal body takes over immediately in the fight for survival; a

◎ traditional japanese nesting dolls consist of a series of dolls of decreasing size; placed one inside another.

skill she will fine tune and put to use way more often than she realizes throughout her womanhood experience. Her body begins to search... *Who can I trust? Am I safe here? Where are my lifelines?*

Regardless of the baby's gender, current rituals around birth in the USA are generally based on hospital procedures and protocol rather than the overall wellbeing of each individual mother and baby. The long-term effects on our nervous systems as an entire culture are not considered in the typical labor and delivery room. As a result, we are experiencing a culture with chronic illness, anxiety and depression at alarming rates - especially in women. ⊚

Could the dishonoring of our very first sacred rite of passage truly play a role in our overall well being? How can we reclaim the power within this passage that we all have a 'rite' to?

⊚ (temkin et al.)

THE BIRTH OF YOU
your first rite of passage

Some things to consider about your own
birth experience, should you have access
to the details of your story:

◎ Who was present at your birth?

◎ Were you forcefully removed from your mother's womb?

◎ Were you separated from your parents at birth?

◎ Were you placed skin-to-skin to learn about the world from
your mother's chest?

◎ Were the lights bright? People shouting? Or was it calm and
inviting?

Some things to consider now:

◎ Have you experienced chronic illnesses, anxiety, depression, or
other symptoms for long periods of time?

◎ Can you have healthy attachment styles in your relationships?
Trust?

◎ Is your nervous system constantly in a state of 'hyperactivity'
or 'overload'?

◎ What have your other sacred rites of passage experiences been
like, such as menarche or entering motherhood? (We'll cover
this more in depth throughout the book.)

III

the wheel of the woman

"midwifery care©
at the center is not only about
pregnancy and birth; but also about
strengthening the family
through creating a welcoming
environment and through
broader health and well-being
programming offered."
-robbie davis floyd; phd

© stemming from old english; the word midwife directly translates to 'with
woman'. this is not limited to support through pregnancy and birth.

An Honor System

Women have always been healers.

Women's traditions for healing date back as far as 'herstory' can recall, and every one of our ancestors had their own magic. One of my favorite her-stories is the tradition of the Appalachian 'Granny' Midwives & Witches. Their lineage dates back to the first Scottish and Irish settlers of the Appalachian Mountains in the 1700s. They blended their own 'old age' traditions with the local tradition of the Cherokee tribes, creating a combination of local folk remedies, faith-based healing, and storytelling.

The Appalachian Granny Traditional Midwives were wise and experienced women who had a deep understanding of herbal remedies and childbirth. They provided medical care and advice to pregnant women and their families, often in the home. They were also responsible for providing spiritual guidance including prayers, blessings, and special ceremonies. The Wise Women and Crones of the community were highly honored and considered the most magical. They were often primarily skilled in midwifery and physical healing, while some of the Appalachian Grannies focused on the power of energetic healing. These traditions have been passed down through generations and remain an important part of the culture in the Appalachian region.

My personal experiences as Woman have brought me to the altar of postmodern methods for healing. Simply put, postmodernism questions current cultural norms. We are challenging the idea that modern influence and interventions on nature are universally beneficial, and reapplying some of our ancestors' wisdom to our modern ways. Less simply put, postmodernism is an Honor System. A postmodern lifestyle is a life of honoring what always has been and what always will be, amidst the currents of constant change.

to understand woman
we must understand
mother nature.
as above; so below.
as within; so without.

In this book we'll continue to explore the inner workings of Woman, first by putting Woman at the center, and then by acknowledging what's around her. This is her true nature.

the wheel of the woman

the earth's rhythm

the sun cycle

woman

the moon cycle

IV

WOMAN
at the center

working with women
allows us to reach the entire
family unit; the entire community.
our 'woman-at-the-center' approach
allows our mission to ripple
throughout households and lineages.

You. At the center. I know you, Woman. You're always caretaking, always tending to the needs of your loved ones. To be in service to Mother Nature and her kin, Woman must first be in service to herself.

Your views on a woman's worthiness are founded on the value you place upon yourself. *Perhaps, this is, in fact, Eve's curse.* The way a woman is treated during her Rites of Passage in life often form her ideas of worthiness and self-value. These images of self then contribute to our values and perceptions of our own worthiness; who we are in this macrosystem. It's time to place yourself at the center, and prioritize your own well being. This is actually a prerequisite to caring for others in a sustainable way.

Inanna's Rite of Passage

The tale of Inanna's descent into the underworld is an ancient myth, woven into the tapestry of human history. Its threads have been spun and respun, each time unearthing new facets of the story's magic. It is a tale of transformation, of traversing the shadows to emerge anew, a story of hope for the women who dare to brave the abyss of their true nature. Her story is a reflection of the cyclical nature of existence, a reminder that every end is a beginning, and every beginning, an end.

In the myth, Inanna, the goddess of love, fertility, and war, decides to descend into the underworld, some say to visit her sister, some say to give birth, some say to find herself.

Regardless of her reasoning, Inanna's journey is a perilous one, and she must pass through seven gates, each of which requires her to remove a piece of her clothing or jewelry, the armor that shields her soul. When she finally reaches her destination, she is naked and vulnerable.

There are many different tales of what Inanna endured while on her journey, but in the end she emerges from the underworld, reborn and renewed, and the world is once again filled with life and fertility.

The story of Inanna's descent into the underworld is a representation of a rite of passage. Like Inanna, a woman must pass through a series of gates, each one more difficult than the last, before she can give birth or be reborn herself. And like Inanna, a woman must surrender herself completely to the process, stripping away that which serves her ego, to face her own vulnerability and mortality. Like Inanna, Woman emerges from the journey stronger, wiser, and filled with more life to give.

EXPLORING
your own rites of passage

Reclaiming our rites of passage takes a new set of rituals- a rebirth. When we tune into the body's symptoms as signs, and use these signs as clues to find 'root causes', we can create healing. There are many ways you can do this- there are no rules. Let's explore.

◎ birth of self (a recap)

Your entrance into this world teaches you about safety, trust, and boundaries.

- Were you forcefully removed from your mother's womb?
- Were you separated from your parents at birth?
- Were you placed skin-to-skin to learn about the world from your mother's chest?
- Were the lights loud? People shouting? Or was it calm and inviting?

◎ childhood to menses

Your beginning years teach you about your place in the world.

- Were your basic needs met?
- Did someone come for and comfort you when you cried?
- Were you given opportunities to make choices and build autonomy?
- Was your first menstruation celebrated and honored? Or hushed and pushed aside?

◎ maiden to mother

Your maiden years teach you about who you are through exploration and self expression.

- Were you given space to explore hobbies and communities?
- Did you have time for your own needs and desires?
- Was the choice 'made for you' to grow up or take on a mother role?
- Were you sexually honored?

◎ birth of each child or creative 'baby'

Your mothering years teach you about your resilience and capacity to love. There are many ways women enter into the 'mother' role. This could be from the birth of a child, an idea, a project, book, business, etc.

- Were your birth experiences or transitions traumatic?
- Was your voice honored and heard during your pregnancies and/or creative 'gestations'?
- Were you cared for and nourished during your postpartum periods?
- Were your mothering skills and instincts trusted and nurtured?

◎ mother to wise woman

This transition is marked by the end of menstruation and brings us back home to ourselves.

- Was there a healthy transition phase to 'empty nesting' or less responsibilities?
- Were the changing hormones in your body honored?
- Did you have a sense of worthiness and value in your community?
- Were you given space to do things you did not have time for as a mother?

◎ death

The End of life season teaches us about the life cycle and our legacy we leave behind.

- Will you be supported by loved ones during your end-of-life time?
- Will your desires about end-of-life care be honored and respected?
- Do you have a sense of completion for your life's work?
- Have you made peace with the end of life and prepared yourself for this transition?

V

earth's
RHYTHM

"Every nature-based culture, from the ancient Celtic people in the Northern hemisphere to the Aboriginal people in the Southern hemisphere, celebrated and marked the cyclic wheel of the year. We need to remember our roots, as they continue to affect us today."
—Lisa Lister, *Witch*

aug 1
lammas

june 20-22
summer
solstice

sept 20-22
fall
equinox

the
wheel of the
year

may 1
beltane

nov 1
samhain

mar 20-22
spring
equinox

dec 20-22
winter
solstice

feb 1
imbolc

Northern Hemisphere

The Celtic Wheel of the Year serves as nature's compass, guiding us with the pulses of the earth's natural cadence. If we choose to dance in sync with these primal rhythms, we befriend the energies of each season and move in unison with them. As the wheel turns, we awaken our feminine intuitive senses to weave a tapestry of flow and harmony that we get to pass down through our lineage.

A Journey through The Sabbats of the Northern Hemisphere

The sabbats on the Wheel of the Year are like nature's own holiday calendar, celebrating the changing seasons. The festivals are marked, renamed and celebrated by cultures all around the world. The traditions surrounding sabbats have been passed down through generations as folklore, and they vary depending on the specific tradition or culture.

Solstice and equinox sabbats are astronomical events, called Solar Festivals, that mark the peak of the seasons. The summer solstice, which occurs around June 20th or 21st in the Northern Hemisphere, marks the longest day of the year and the official peak of summer. The winter solstice, which falls on December 21st or 22nd, is the shortest day of the year and marks the peak of winter.

Equinoxes occur when the Earth's tilt is such that the day and night are of equal length.

The spring equinox occurs on March 20th or 21st and marks the official peak of spring in the Northern Hemisphere. The fall equinox, which falls on September 22nd or 23rd, marks the peak of autumn.

In between the solstices and equinoxes, the ancestors celebrate the Fire festivals (Samhain, Imbolc, Beltane, and Lammas). These sabbats mark a transition point, the endings and beginnings of each season, if you will. While exploring what importances our ancestors placed on these seasons, you may notice similarities to our modern day Gregorian calendar holidays as you get to the core origins of our common cultural traditions.

*Note that the sabbats of the Southern Hemisphere are opposite, to match up with their seasonal rotation.
Example: The Winter Solstice is in June and the Summer Solstice is in December for the Southern Hemisphere.

SAMHAIN

samhain falls on november 1st; marking
the midway point between the fall
equinox and the winter solstice.
this is the entrance into the dark season.

NOVEMBER 1

Samhain (pronounced "SAH-win") is a season to savor your harvest and connect with ancestral wisdom by honoring your passed relatives and loved ones. It is believed that during this time, the veil between the world of the living and the world of the dead is at its thinnest, allowing spirits to reconnect and share messages with one another. Our ancestors had different rituals surrounding this time to call upon those who came before them. These traditions have been passed down and turned into celebrations you may recognize today, like Halloween, Día de los Muertos and All Saints Day.

APPLYING
samhain to your season

◉ create an ancestors altar.

If you don't have a seasonal altar in your home, now is the time to make one! It can be simple and small enough to fit into a box if you have a small space, or you can make it an elaborate work of art that constantly evolves and changes with the seasons. Around Samhain, decorate your seasonal altar to honor your ancestors, similarly to Día De Los Muertos traditions. You can include photos and keepsakes from your loved ones that have passed on, certain foods/scents that remind you of them, letters, flowers, etc.

◉ have a bonfire ceremony.

Ready to release the shit in life that's holding you back? Nature and the trees show us how to effortlessly release each cycle's beauty to make room for what is next. Forests could not grow without destruction. Start a bonfire, burn a letter listing what you are releasing, and embrace the season of introspection and reflection. (Be sure to practice fire safety!)

◎ host a 'silent supper' for grief support.

Invite friends that are grieving or host your own private silent supper, setting places at the table for your passed loved ones. Begin with a moment of silence, have a toast to your ancestors and share your favorite memories of your 'silent supper' guests of honor for laughs and maybe a few tears.

◎ reflect on your year.

In our busy culture, it's easy to skip over reflections and celebrations to start reaching towards the 'next big thing'. Samhain is the time to go through journal entries, take inventory of what you have learned, how you have grown, and what new wisdom you have accumulated.

◎ plan for the next journey around the wheel of the year.

Samhain is the season of introspection, serving as the first piece of your guide to the year ahead. We don't just wake up one day totally different, it's a process of intentionally moving through the slow seasons. Now is a good time to review your intentions and maybe even try a Wheel of the Year tarot or oracle spread, *if you're into that sorta thing*!

wheel of the year
AHEAD SPREAD

How to do a Wheel of the Year Card Spread

Set a sacred scene, connect with your deck, and ask for guidance
on your coming year. When you're ready, draw eight cards and set
them in a circle, representing the Wheel of the Year. Finally, draw
a 9th card to place in the middle of the wheel. Spend time
examining the imagery on each card, and note any intuitive
messages you are receiving. If you want more information, you can
always turn to the deck's guidebook for more guidance.

- Card One: A Message for Samhain (Current)
- Card Two: A Message for Yule
- Card Three: A Message for Imbolc
- Card Four: A Message for Ostara
- Card Five: A Message for Beltane
- Card Six: A Message for Litha
- Card Seven: A Message for Lammas
- Card Eight: A Message for Mabon
- Card Nine: An Insight on your Overall Year Ahead

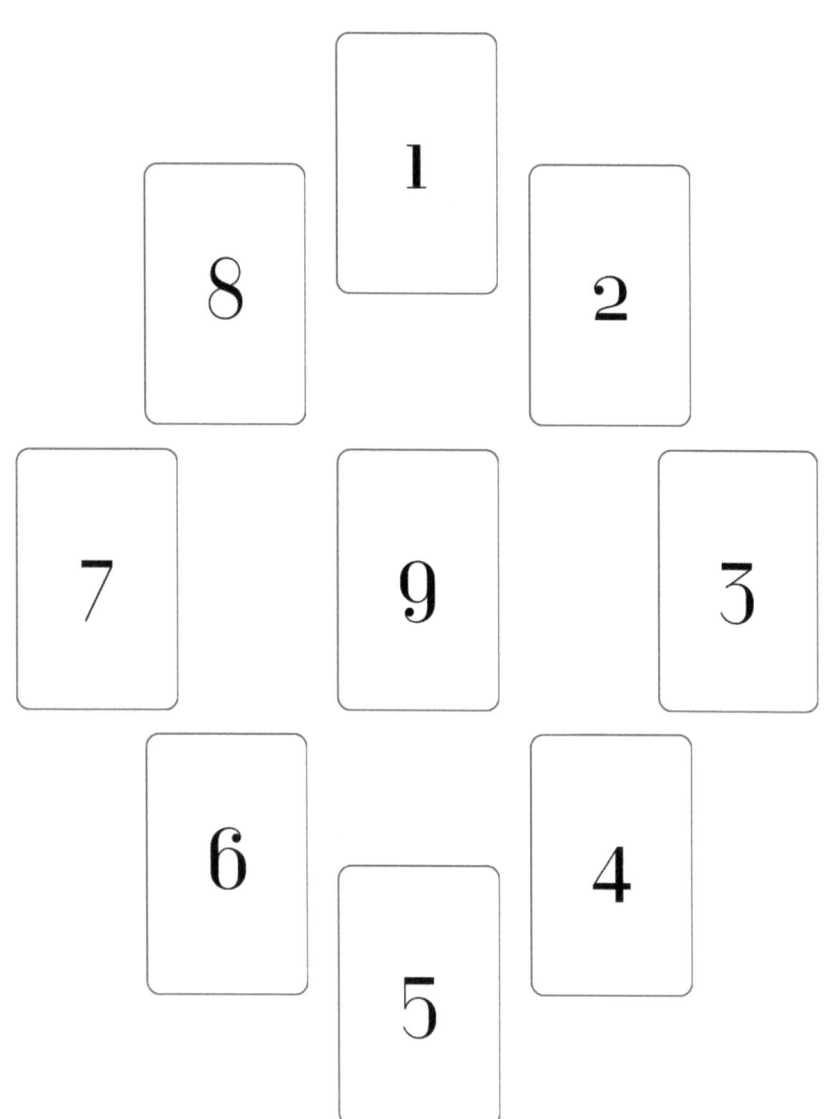

YULE

WINTER SOLSTICE

winter solstice falls around december 21st;
marking the darkest day of the year.
this is the peak of winter.

DECEMBER 21

On or around December 21st, the sun pauses, and then changes direction.® This marks the solstice, or Yule, as it's called on the Wheel of the Year. This is like the Sun's Rebirth. While the immediate days to come are still short, we are at the tipping point of the Wheel. The shift in directions is upon us.

There's a fascinating Scandinavian Yule story that has lived on so strongly, you may recognize it. According to passed down folktale, during the long winter months, there were highly respected shamans that delivered the present of presence with a mystical touch. These shaman would journey over the high snows in a sleigh (pulled by reindeer, of course) collecting and distributing little red and white gifts that grow under the evergreen pine trees - the amanita muscaria. I can imagine that hunkering down for the winter could be an isolating and boring season for our ancestors, so the relief that these little gifts brought probably made these little magical shaman pretty popular. They may even show their gratitude by leaving him a little sweet treat.

APPLYING
yule to your season

◎ **focus on nourishment.**

Now is the time to nourish in preparation for spring, rather than succumbing to the 'New Year, New Me' culture in the middle of winter. Keep the fire burning and fan your creative flames in the kitchen with soup recipes and herbal teas.

◎ **create a hygge home for positive mental health.**

Hygge is a Danish word that has no direct English translation, but it refers to a feeling of coziness, comfort, and warmth that promotes a sense of well-being and contentment. Studies show that the Danes are the happiest people in the world- despite the dark, cold winters that they experience!◎ Create a Hygge home that is tidy but cozy, aesthetically pleasing, and adorned with items that carry stories and bring joy to the people within the walls. For Yule, the whole home is your altar!

◎ **burn a yule log.**

The tradition of the yule log kept our ancestors warm amidst the longest night of the year. They would save a large log of fallen oak to ceremonially burn on the night of the solstice. Revive the tradition by gathering around the fire with your housemates, family or closest friends to share stories, eat, drink, and be merry.

◎ (meik wiking)

◎ bring the evergreens indoors.

Pine trees are called evergreen because they keep their green needles all year round, even during the winter months when most other trees have gone bare. This resilience stems from a deep-rooted adaptation to weather the harshest of elements. Thus, the pine tree serves as a symbol of our own innate strength, a reminder that we too possess the fortitude to flourish in even the harshest of environments. So pick out your evergreen, decorate her, and honor her strength! (Consider a potted pine that can be re-planted after the season passes.)

◎ hang mistletoe as a symbol of peace.

In Norse mythology, mistletoe was seen as a sacred symbol of peace and love, offering healing and protective powers to those who received it. This belief eventually led to the practice of hanging mistletoe in homes during the holiday season as a symbol of love and goodwill.

IMBOLC

imbolc falls on february 1st; marking the
midway point between the winter solstice
and the spring equinox.
the light is returning.

FEBRUARY 1

Imbolc translates roughly to 'in the belly' or 'ewe's milk'. The Earth is pregnant with new life. It's a time that represents hope as winter begins to fade. This day is marked with a festival celebrating Brigid, the Triple Goddess, as she represents the movement from maiden to mother to crone and back again. Brigid is also known as the goddess of poetry, healing, midwifery and smithcraft. She is called upon to usher in new life, abundance, and health as the earth reawakens.

APPLYING
imbolc to your season

◉ let the light in.

There are different rituals you can perform to invite the light back in. If there is snow on the ground, head outside and find a spot in the sun. Draw a picture of the sun into the snow on the ground and stand behind it with your face towards the sun. Call in the light. No sun? Light a candle or flip the switches on in every room of your house at sunset to represent the light lasting a little longer, inviting the light to stay.

◉ honor your rites of passage.

Under the holiday of the Triple Goddess, it's a great time to review your relationship with the Rites of Passage you've experienced thus far, and how they've shaped you. Allow this to be a rebirth, even recreating a sacred rite of passage ceremony if you feel called.

◉ get creative.

Call on Brigid to work through your hands. Try a hobby or craft you've been interested in, particularly one that requires you to use your handcrafting skills, such as painting, pottery, sewing, etc.

◎ practice your poetry.

Poetry allows us to express ourselves in a creative and meaningful way, and can be a powerful tool for self-reflection and growth. Try experimenting with different forms of poetry - haikus, sonnets, free verse - and see what feels most natural to you. Most importantly, have fun!

◎ incorporate kundalini breath of fire into your morning routine.

There are many stories and folklore about the kundalini serpent reawakening around Imbolc. Kundalini yoga is a powerful tool that can help you build strength, increase energy, and enhance your overall wellbeing. One of the core practices in Kundalini yoga is the *Breath of Fire*. This breathing technique stimulates the body and mind, and helps to awaken the Kundalini serpent energy that is said to lie dormant at the base of the spine.

kundalini
BREATH OF FIRE

To practice the Breath of Fire, follow these steps:

- Find a comfortable seated position with your spine straight and your hands resting on your knees.
- Take a deep breath in through your nose, filling your lungs completely.
- Exhale forcefully through your nose, pulling your navel in towards your spine as you do so- it feels similar to blowing your nose.
- Begin to breathe rapidly and rhythmically through your nose, without pausing between inhales and exhales. Keep your focus on pushing your navel out for the exhale. The inhale will happen naturally.
- Practice this breathing technique for 1-3 minutes to start, gradually increasing the duration as you become more comfortable with the practice.

◎ Warning: Breath of Fire is stimulating and is best practiced in the morning, as to not disrupt your sleep pattern. Avoid this practice if you are actively menstruating, pregnant, breastfeeding or ill.

OSTARA

SPRING EQUINOX

spring equinox falls around march 21st;
marking the return of balance.
this is the peak of spring.

MARCH 21

Twelve hours of light, twelve hours of darkness. The Spring Equinox is a renewal, the return of longer days and the warmth of the sun. On the Celtic Wheel of the Year this is also known as Ostara, named after the Germanic goddess of fertility and new beginnings. She's often associated with rabbits, eggs, and spring bulbs such as tulips and daffodils, similar to our modern Easter holiday. In addition, the etymology of Ostara seems to stem from the Anglo-Saxon goddess, *Eostre*.

APPLYING
ostara to your season

◎ incorporate an egg ritual.

Review your visions and goals for this season of growth and then ritualistically place these intentions into an egg. You can simply meditate with the egg in your hands, thinking about what you want to grow in your life, or you can decorate the egg with symbolic representations. Then bury the egg in the soil of your garden, intentionally planting your goals into the darkness so they can grow towards the light. Use this as fertilizer for a rose bush or a plant that is special to you.

◎ plant a bulb garden.

Start planting a bulb garden (try tulips or daffodils), representing the creative flowers that will bloom in your life this year. Choose a location with plenty of sunlight and well-draining soil. Plant bulbs at a depth that is two to three times their height, space them evenly, and water well. The bulbs will remain dormant until the weather warms up and then watch your creative babies bloom. With proper care and planning, you can have a beautiful bulb garden for years to come that you tend to every Spring Equinox. Already have a bulb garden? Tend to it now, remove dead foliage and debris, fertilize the soil, separate bulbs that are too close, and give them some love.

◎ try a milk and honey tradition.

Milk and honey are believed to symbolize purity, renewal, and new beginnings, which are all central themes of the equinox. In some cultures, they start the day off with a sweet combination of milk and honey, a tradition that embodies the hope and promise of new beginnings. Other traditions include mixing the two into sweet honey cakes and pastries, or anointing the body with sacred milk and honey blends.

◎ spring cleaning time!

Dust away the winter cobwebs- physically and figuratively. Declutter, reorganize, and deep clean your sacred spaces. In addition to cleaning your physical spaces, reassess your mental and emotional health. Take some time to reflect on how you've been feeling. Begin to reincorporate a healthy habit that may have slipped away with the darkness. By taking care of your home and yourself, you'll be ready to welcome the new season with a fresh start.

◎ make a besom.

A besom is a broom made of natural materials used to ritualistically sweep away the literal and figurative cobwebs.

make your own
BESOM

- Find a sturdy wooden stick or branch about 3-4 feet long. This will be the handle of your besom.
- Collect a bundle of fresh herbs, such as rosemary, lavender, or sage. These herbs are often associated with purification and renewal, making them perfect for a Spring Equinox besom.
- Tie the herbs to the end of the wooden stick using natural twine or string. Make sure the herbs are tightly secured to the stick.
- Gather a small bundle of dried straw or hay. This will be the bristles of your besom.
- Using the same twine or string, tie the straw or hay to the bottom of the wooden stick. Make sure the bristles are evenly distributed and tightly secured to the stick.
- Trim any excess twine or string and your besom is complete.
- Time to sweep!

BELTANE

beltane falls on may 1st; marking the
midway point between the spring
equinox and the summer solstice.
this is the entrance into the light season.

MAY 1

The Beltane fire festival fans the flames of creativity and fertility. Nature is full of vitality and growth at this time, and so are we. It is said that this is a time to connect with the spirits of nature, to celebrate the earthly experience of being human. We can take part in the sacred celebration of Beltane simply by reconnecting with Mother Nature and her children (plants, animals, humans, etc)

APPLYING
beltane to your season

◎ move your body.

Beltane is a great time to let loose. If you have a partner, this is a great time to spice things up and celebrate the spark that you tended into a flame. If you're currently single, reconnect with your body through sacred pleasure practices or movement that brings you joy. Now's the time to try that belly dancing or pole class you've been eyeing to get your sacral energies moving.

◎ host a maypole festival.

One of the most beloved traditions of Beltane is the dance around the maypole. The community comes together around a pole, holding ribbons attached to the top of the pole, weaving in and out of each other with every step they take. The ribbons create a stunning pattern, making for a beautiful visual display, and symbolizing the interconnectedness of all of us in nature.

◎ try weaving.

Whether you make a basket, weave a tapestry, or simply braid sweetgrass you can creatively symbolize the flow between masculinity and femininity that we celebrate during Beltane season.

◎ visit a body of water.

Head to a pond, lake, stream, river or shoreline to admire the beauty of nature's pools. You can ceremonially swim in the water, send a flower mandala down the stream, or just dip a toe and say a gratitude prayer.

◎ make a fire with the nine sacred woods.

Each type of wood on the Beltane fire represents different aspects of the natural world, and lighting the fire symbolizes the alchemy of the elements for the creation of something new. There are many variations of the 'Nine Sacred Woods' from different sources. *Remember, intention is everything.* This list is from Lisa Lister's book, *Witch.*

1. Birch: purification
2. Rowan: spiritual protection
3. Ash: strength, renewal
4. Elder: balance of earth and water
5. Willow: intuitive guidance
6. Hawthorn: protection of hearth and home
7. Oak: ancestral wisdom
8. Holly: balance of darkness and light
9. Yew: longevity, rebirth

LITHA
SUMMER SOLSTICE

summer solstice falls around june 21st;
marking the lightest day of the year.
this is the peak of summer.

JUNE 21

More widely known as the Summer Solstice, on the Wheel of the Year the lightest day of the year is marked as Litha. On this day, the sun is at its highest point in the sky, and the hours of daylight are the longest they will be all year, fulfilling the promise of the evergreen cycle, that the light always returns. It is a time to rejoice in the strength you have found within yourself to make it to this point, and also a time to refuel with the power of the sun to finish out the harvest.

Traditionally, Litha is celebrated with bonfires, feasting, and dancing. It is a time to come together with friends and family, to celebrate the warmth and light of the sun, and to give thanks for all the blessings in our lives. This is similar to the rituals our culture practices at the exact *opposite* point on the wheel of the year.

APPLYING
litha to your season

◎ soak up the sun.

Schedule in time to watch the sunrise and sunset on these long summer days, honoring the extended hours of light and giving gratitude for all of the blessings and beauty of the sun.

◎ honor the sambucus harvest.

Now is the true time to eat, drink and be merry! Elderberry and elderflower both come from the sambucus plant. You can try making elderflower champagne to share with your friends or connect with the spirits of your elders, and use the elderberries to make healing medicines and syrups to boost the immune system and reduce inflammation.

◎ revisit your vows.

In the Litha spirit of promises, strength and never ending cycles- now is the time to revisit and possibly even recreate your vows- to your partner or family, to your dreams, to yourself. Never written vows to yourself before? You can write yourself a love letter, of promises to protect and prioritize yourself. Maybe even recite these vows in front of a mirror or a close group of friends to declare your commitment.

◎ start a dream journal.

The pique of summer is the time for those *midsummer night dreams*. Keep a dream journal nearby so that you can capture the magic of your psyche under the light Litha skies. You can also place a pouch of dried mugwort and bay leaves under your pillow to enhance your dreams!

◎ do your sun salutations.

In yogic traditions, Sun Salutations are a foundational practice that cultivate a sense of inner strength, while honoring and giving thanks for the solar power from the sun that fuels our gardens, our bodies, and all living things.

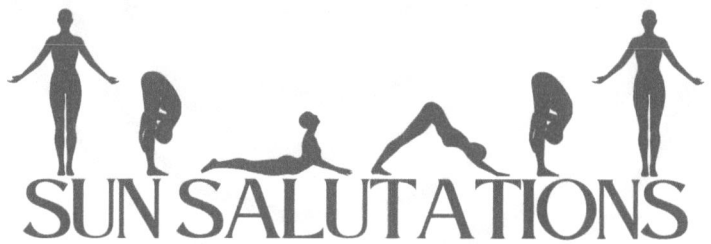

SUN SALUTATIONS

- Start by standing at the top of your mat with your feet hips-distance apart and your hands at heart center. Take a few breaths, pushing into all four corners of your feet, grounding into the body and your practice.
- Inhale, as you reach up, bringing your arms and gaze upward.
- Exhale, folding forward.
- Inhale, bringing your hands to the shins, and lifting up to a straight spine.
- Exhale, lowering your hands back down to the ground, and stepping back to plank pose.
- Inhale, rolling onto your tip-toes bringing your heart forward.
- Exhale, lowering down to the ground in one line of energy.
- Inhale, pushing into the hands and pulling your heart forward and up into a cobra pose.
- Exhale, rolling over the toes and pushing back into downward facing dog.
- Inhale, shifting to the tip-toes, as you bend the knees, and look towards the front of the mat.
- Exhale, stepping your feet back to the top of the mat into a forward fold.
- Repeat the sequence. For a full Sun Salute ritual, some will do this practice 108 times in a row.

LAMMAS

lammas falls on august 1st; marking the midway point between the summer solstice and the fall equinox.
the harvest is coming.

AUGUST 1

Lammas, also known as Lughnasadh, is a fire festival that marks the beginning of the harvest season. The name Lammas comes from the Old English word "hlafmaesse," meaning "loaf mass." During this time, people would bake bread from the first grains of the harvest, sharing as a blessing for more to come. Then, they feast!

In Celtic mythology, Lammas was associated with the god Lugh, who was a master of many skills, including agriculture. The festival was a time to honor his role in the harvest and to thank the gods for their bounty.

APPLYING
lammas to your season

◎ bake bread!

Connect with the Earth and honor the farmers who bring in the first crops of the year by putting it to use in your creative kitchen. Use grains or seeds harvested at this time, add dried fruit, nuts, or herbs, and think about the hard work that goes into growing and harvesting. Give thanks for the Earth's abundance and nourishment, and share your bread with friends and family.

◎ incorporate a gratitude ritual into your daily routine.

While we could benefit from gratitude rituals all the time, it can be particularly powerful to take a moment each day during this season to reflect on the blessings in your life and give thanks for them. You can do this through prayer, meditation, or simply by intentionally and authentically expressing your gratitude to those around you.

◎ work with herbs.

A *Wise Woman* tradition is to incorporate harvested and dried herbs into your festivities. Herbs such as chamomile, lavender, and thyme are all associated with this holiday and can be used to create teas, tinctures, and other herbal remedies. You can also create an herbal wreath or bouquet to decorate your home or altar.

◎ make a corn dolly.

Harvest season brings out the corn dolls, made from those papery corn husks. These cuties aren't just a pretty sight; they're also like little guardians against bad juju. Many cultures believe in their magical mojo, so they pop them in their homes as a talisman for happy vibes.

◎ host a gratitude circle.

Have your Friendsgiving 'early' according to our culture. Now is a great time to heed the harvest and break bread with your favorite folks. It's a perfect way to kick off the harvest season, and reap the benefits of seasonal living in community. Want to make it more sacred? You can get creative with my basic outline for a Gratitude Circle.

hosting a
GRATITUDE CIRCLE

An intentional gathering with your local friends can be a perfect way to celebrate sacred bonds, and can serve to strengthen the spiritual connection between the folks in your community.

- Begin the gathering with a meditation circle and bring awareness to the gratitude filling the room for one another. You can use calming music or guided meditations to help set the tone.
- After meditation, prompt everyone in the room to take a few minutes to write down what they are grateful for in their friendships. This exercise can help deepen the appreciation for one another.
- Once everyone has had a chance to journal, come together in a sharing circle. Each person can share their thoughts, feelings, and experiences on friendship. This exercise can be an excellent opportunity to learn more about each other and the bonds that exist between you. It may also be a space to heal wounds from past friendships and experiences.
- End the gathering with a blessing ceremony and feast. You can light candles and offer sweet sentiments to each other over a bottle of wine or mocktails.

MABON

FALL EQUINOX

fall equinox falls around september 21st;
marking the return of balance.
this is the peak of autumn.

SEPTEMBER 21

The fall equinox, also known as Mabon, is a return to balance, a turning point back towards the darker half of the wheel. It is a time to celebrate the abundance of the previous months and to prepare for the coming winter. Once again, we experience twelve hours of light, twelve hours of darkness.

APPLYING
mabon to your season

◉ pumpkin spice it up.

I know that the popular pumpkin spice trend is a hit or miss, but it's one of the seasonal celebrations that we largely partake in as a culture, so I'm calling it a win! Pumpkins, squash, and root vegetables are harvested at this time, and they make great ingredients in the kitchen, decorations on the altar, and even tools for your crafts. Pick your perfect pumpkin from your garden or the local patch and get creative to use every bit of it.

◉ thank a local farmer.

This is the farmer's favorite season! Head to a local apple orchard, pumpkin patch, or farmer's market and celebrate the hard work of your local farmers by visiting, supporting, buying, and giving gratitude.

◉ preserve your harvest.

One of the main traditions associated with Mabon is the preservation of the harvest. To practice preserving your harvest, you can try drying or pickling some seasonal produce or take your shot at making jams and jellies. You could even prepare to stay warm through the winter with your own homemade cider and mead.

◎ take an autumn nature walk.

Explore the beauty of the equinox and the changes that come with it. Take deep breaths as you walk, taking in the crisp autumn air. The leaves are starting to change color and fall from their branches, creating a beautiful carpet of red, orange, and yellow beneath our feet. Keep an eye out for the different animals that call this space home. Maybe squirrels are busy gathering nuts, birds are migrating south, and deer are courting for mating season. There is so much activity happening in the natural world during this time of year. Notice the transition taking place from summer to winter and bask in the beauty of nature's cycles.

◎ host a harvest potluck.

Heed the harvest and celebrate with friends by bringing everyone together with their own contributions. Enjoy each other's creations and share the year's accomplishments with one another.

VI

moon CYCLES

unraveling the web of
women's health issues
really starts with examining
our cultural beliefs
and expectations on women
to uphold a linear lifestyle
within a cyclical design.

This is where you're going to start to see the intricate connections that weave the web of Woman. Your menstrual cycle, which is 28-ish days long for most women, is your personal moon cycle. Our body is constantly attempting to mimic the moon's 28-ish day cycle, giving us information via our Fifth Vital Sign, as Lisa Hendrickson-Jack has coined it.[©] Our society has a pretty linear point of view, male or female. In the good ol' USA, most working women get *zero* chill time for Aunt Flo's visits or our hormonal ups and downs. So, we're often left feeling like we have no choice but to power through, chug caffeine (which can be a real adrenal drag during that time of the month), and keep on shining.

Throughout history, there were many different ways that cultures viewed women's cycles. Some viewed women as dirty and unholy during her bleed, while others honored the cycle with Red Tent traditions.

Red Tents were sanctuaries where women would retreat during their menstrual cycles. It was common for most women of the village to bleed *together*, in alignment with the moon cycles. *This has changed since modern women often use hormonal contraceptives and/or have dysregulated circadian rhythms from late nights under fluorescent lights.* These sacred red tent spaces provided community support and rejuvenation for our ancestors that experienced them.

Women would gather to share their experiences, knowledge, and wisdom, passing it down from generation to generation while weaving magic into one another's braids. (That's how I picture it, anyways.) As time went on, the significance of red tents evolved. In some lineages, they became spaces for childbirth and postpartum recovery. Women would come together, offering support and assistance throughout the birthing process, ensuring the well-being of both mother and child. The passing down of these midwifery-like rituals slowed as the Industrial Revolution called women into the modern workforce, away from their body's natural cycles and rhythms.

Today, the concept of red tents is being reimagined and revitalized. It has become a symbol for reclaiming feminine power and celebrating the sacredness of womanhood. Red tent gatherings and workshops have emerged as spaces for women to connect, share, and grow together, creating a sense of sisterhood and empowerment. The history of red tents continues to inspire and reshape the way we perceive and honor the experiences of women.

Each moon cycle is a mini representation of a season, a rite of passage, an opportunity to retell your story and strengthen your narrative.

ovulation
full moon

luteal
**waning
moon**

menstrual
moon cycles

follicular
**waxing
moon**

the bleed
**new
moon**

understanding your moon cycle

menstrual phase	moon phase	season	rite of passage
Follicular	Waxing Moon	Spring	Maiden
Ovulation	Full Moon	Summer	Mother
Luteal	Waning Moon	Fall	Wise Woman
Menstruation	New Moon	Winter	Death/Rebirth

*Note: If you are not a menstruating woman, you can use the moon herself as your guide to tuning into the moon cycles.

Follicular

Bleeding has just subsided, estrogen is increasing, and creativity is building.

The follicular phase is the spring of your moon cycle. During this phase, the body gets creative, developing follicles in the ovaries. As these follicles grow, estrogen is produced, causing the lining of the uterus to thicken, preparing for a potential pregnancy.

The energy of the waxing moon is generally associated with growth and expansion. As the moon moves from new towards full, its light and energy are said to be increasing. This is a time to focus on setting intentions, making plans, and taking action toward goals.

Ovulation

Estrogen piques, an egg is released, and sacral energy is at its fullest.

The ovulation phase is the summer of your moon cycle. Estrogen levels pique, leading to an increase in energy, clarity, and sexual desire. It's a great time to tackle new projects, try new things, collaborate and connect. It's also the time to get intimate if you're wanting to conceive, or be extra careful if that's not the goal!

The full moon is often associated with mystery and magic. She causes pendulums to swing with her bright and powerful forces. Tides flow from their highest to lowest, emotions are felt at their fullest expressions, and whatever we have been focusing on becomes amplified. It is believed that during this time, the veil between the physical and spiritual worlds is thin, making it easier to connect with our ancestors, guides, and gods. It's go time!

Luteal

Progesterone piques, heavier emotions resurface, and creative output diminishes.

During this phase, the ruptured follicle that released the egg transforms into a structure called the corpus luteum. The corpus luteum secretes progesterone, which helps prepare the uterus for potential pregnancy by thickening the uterine lining.

The waning moon asks us to move inward again, recognizing and unraveling another layer of Woman. Focus on rest and rejuvenation. As the moon's energy decreases, it is a good time to slow down, sip tea, and go back to the basics of nurturing Woman first.

Menstruation
Uterine lining sheds, menstruation begins, Woman rebirths.

If your hormonal cycle was a season, menstruation would be winter. While on your period (or moon time), you might have a stronger desire to rest, indulge in comfort, and skip your HIIT workout for the week. Instead of hitting the gym, try a creative release such as painting, cooking, or a restorative yoga class.

The dark moon, also known as the new moon, is the phase of the moon when it is not visible from the Earth. During this time, the moon is positioned between the Earth and the Sun, essentially blocking out the light of the Sun, leaving only the dark side of the moon visible to us.

This is a time for hibernation and restorative preparations. It is an opportunity to release that which holds you back with a new awareness of a deeper layer of Woman.

If you are looking to make changes in your life or to connect more deeply with your inner self, the dark moon is a powerful time to do so.

honoring your
MOON CYCLE

- **Food as Medicine.**

For healthier cycles that are less symptomatic, try filling your plate with high quality animal proteins, organic produce and fermented foods. Pairing your sugar/carbs with a protein will help balance blood sugar and maintain energy levels, while the fermented foods will help cultivate a healthy gut biome! QUALITY MATTERS. Go for local, grass-fed, pasture-raised, organic - all the things - whenever possible.

- **Limit Artificial Light Exposure.**

Artificial lights have an effect on our hormones, sleep patterns and overall wellness. Limiting light exposure when the sun is not out can help keep you attuned to the circadian rhythm and even shorten menstruation time.

◎ *Other ways to Regulate your Circadian Rhythm:*
  - Sleep in a completely dark space (or wear an eye mask!)
  - Minimize blue light exposure (phone/tv/computer) at night. You can also invest in some blue-light blocking glasses if you work late to minimize the impact.
  - Let the sunrise hit your eyes. The early morning sun resets the internal clock, giving a boost of energy for the day and improving sleep at night.

- Limit caffeine consumption. Try a mushroom or herbal based coffee alternative, and avoid caffeine altogether after 3 pm if possible.
- Move your body. Daily exercise and movement allows the body to rest better at night (P.S. Studies show that sex before bed promotes better sleep, too.)

- **Prioritize emotional well-being.**

Your body is an intricate system designed to aid in your human experience. When you tune into the emotions that arise during the physical process of releasing (menstruation), you create space for deeper healing (health). Slow down and listen.

◎ *Healthy Ways to Prioritize your Emotions:*
- Practice mindfulness or meditation. You can find a local class, try a YouTube video, or try a creative meditation such as painting.
- Reconnect with old passions. Play music, make art, sing.
- Spend time in nature.
- Journal. Allow your emotions to flow out of you and onto the page. (Burn it after, if you want! Practice fire safety- of course.)

- **Let the Blood Flow.**

Consider switching to organic pads or reusable period products to limit your toxin exposure and send your body the message that it's okay to slow down and honor this process.

"Anecdotally, many women who've replaced their regular pads and tampons with organic versions (or reusable versions such as menstrual cups and cloth pads) experience a significant decrease in menstrual cramping and other menstrual cycle issues."
    -Lisa Hendrickson-Jack, The Fifth Vital Sign

- **Track your cycle.**

The Fertility Awareness Method is the formula to understanding your Fifth Vital Sign. There are three main bodily functions that we can track to determine our fertile window: *cervical mucus, basal body temperature, and cervical position.*

   - Cervical mucus is a fluid produced by the cervix that changes in consistency and texture throughout the menstrual cycle. During ovulation, cervical mucus becomes thinner and more stretchy, resembling egg whites. This type of cervical mucus helps sperm swim through the cervix and into the uterus to fertilize an egg.

   - Basal body temperature (BBT) is the body's resting temperature, which can be measured orally or vaginally using a special thermometer. BBT tends to rise by about 0.5 to 1 degree Fahrenheit after ovulation and remains elevated until the next menstrual period. By tracking your BBT over time, you can identify patterns in your menstrual cycle and predict when ovulation might occur.

- Cervical position refers to the position and texture of the cervix itself. During ovulation, the cervix becomes softer, higher, and more open. By becoming familiar with the position of the cervix using your fingers, you can gain insight into your fertility status.

◎ *How is Fertility Awareness (FA) beneficial?*

- For women on a path outside of motherhood, FA can be a method of natural birth control that has an effectiveness rate of up to 99.4%.◎

- For women wishing to conceive, FA allows a woman to understand when she is ovulating for her best chances at fertilizing the egg.

- For women without a cycle, understanding the three bodily functions of FA offers alternative methods to tap into her personal natural rhythm.

- For creative women, the rhythm of creativity that pulses in synchronicity with the body's cycle is a superpower.

- ALL wise women, understanding the health of our cycles can be beneficial to our overall well being.

The only way to develop a deep relationship with your cycle is to establish a daily ritual of checking in on your fertility. Incorporate this into your morning routine. You can track physical symptoms, feelings, and other daily indicators on paper charts or in an app on your phone.

elemental
DAILY
scheduling

If you've been camping, have you ever noticed how your habits shift after a few days in the wilderness? Usually, you get up earlier as the sun rises to warm up, your day gets active a little quicker, and you settle in near a fire at sundown for a little story time before bed. This is probably how our ancestors did it, too. Before the blue lights of televisions, computers, phones, and overhead fluorescent lighting, there were less distractions to pull us away from the day's natural cycle. Nowadays, we have the ability to stay up late doing laundry in the electric dryer, wash dishes with our running hot water, and work on our latest project using our laptops while we catch up on the latest sitcoms until 2 am - all of which has a deep impact on our overall wellbeing overtime.

In an attempt to master the mundane by realigning our daily lives with the daily earth rhythm - the Sun Cycle - we must first understand the basics of *Ayurveda*. Ayurveda is the sister science of yoga, filled with traditions backed by ancient wisdom. The entire philosophy is broken down into three elements, or *doshas*, which serve as a basic guide for all of existence. Each being has a unique balance of these doshas - Vata, Pitta, and Kapha. Vata represents *air*, Pitta represents *fire*, and Kapha represents *earth* and *water*. To align our daily schedules with the sun's cycle, we will break down how these elements are associated with time, and use them as a guide for our day-to-day rituals.

the essence of
THE ELEMENTS

The elements that make up our world are fascinating and essential to life as we know it. From the air we breathe, to the ground beneath our feet, each element plays a crucial role in maintaining the delicate balance of our planet. Fire, water, earth, and air are the fundamental elements that have been recognized since ancient times, and each has unique characteristics and properties.

◎ *Water* is the element of emotion, intuition, and healing. It represents the flow of life and is associated with purification and cleansing.

◎ *Earth* is the element of stability, grounding, and material reality. It represents the physical world and is associated with growth and nurturing.

◎ *Fire* represents energy, passion, and transformation. It is the element of change and is associated with creativity and willpower.

◎ *Air* is the element of thought, communication, and intellect. It represents the power of the mind and is associated with clarity and inspiration.

vata
2 pm - 6 pm

pitta
10 am - 2 pm

kapha
6 pm - 10 pm

ayurvedic
sun cycles

kapha
6 am - 10 am

pitta
10 pm - 2 am

vata
2 am - 6 am

AYURVEDIC SCHEDULING
the elements & time

This is your guide to reconnecting your daily life with the elements of the earth.

grand rising [6 am - 10 am]

- *Element*: earth & water // Kapha
- *Themes*: gratitude & devotion, morning rituals
  - *Prompts*: What am I grateful for? How can I set myself up for success today?

solar power [10 am - 2 pm]

- *Element*: fire // Pitta
- *Themes*: focus, action, productivity
  - *Prompts*: How can I serve/live out my purpose today? How can I fuel my body?

breeze of inspiration [2 pm - 6 pm]

- *Element*: air // Vatta
- *Themes*: creativity, exploration
  - *Prompts*: How can I express myself today? How can I feed my soul?

soak it in [6 pm - 10 pm]

- *Element*: earth & water // Kapha
- *Themes*: integration, evening rituals
  - *Prompts*: How can I express my gratitude? How can I set myself up for success tomorrow?

rest & restore [10 pm - 2 am]

- *Element*: fire // Pitta
- *Themes*: digestion, restoration
  - *Prompts*: Keep a tidy & sacred sleep space. Have a consistent bedtime routine. Limit late night snacking and blue light exposure. Apply topical magnesium before bed.

dream state [2 am - 6 am]

- *Element*: air // Vatta
- *Themes*: dreams, spiritual integration
  - *Prompts*: Take at least 1 day off a week from herbal sleep aids. Limit daily caffeine intake. Keep a dream altar and journal by the bed.

VIII

the wheel of the woman
NOTES

BIBLIOGRAPHY
& many thanks

Davis-Floyd, Robbie, et al. Birth Models That Work. Berkeley, University Of California Press, Cop, 2009.

Gaherty, Geoff. "Winter Solstice: The Sun Stands Still on Saturday." Space.com, 18 Dec. 2013, www.space.com/24014-winter-solstice-sun-movement-explained.html.

Hendrickson-Jack, Lisa, and Lara Briden. The Fifth Vital Sign : Master Your Cycles and Optimize Your Fertility. Fertility Friday Publishing Inc, 2019.

Lister, Lisa. Witch. Carlsbad, California, Hay House, 2017.

Palma, Cosimo. "The Etymology of "Woman" in Different Languages | Terminology Coordination Unit." Terminology Coordination, 30 July 2019, termcoord.eu/2019/07/the-etimology-of-woman-in-different-languages/.

Temkin, Sarah M., et al. "Chronic Conditions in Women: The Development of a National Institutes of Health Framework." BMC Women's Health, vol. 23, no. 1, 6 Apr. 2023, https://doi.org/10.1186/s12905-023-02319-x.

Watterson, Meggan. MARY MAGDALENE REVEALED : The First Apostle, Her Feminist Gospel & the Christianity We Haven't... Tried Yet. S.L., Hay House Inc, 2020.

Wiking, Meik. The Little Book of Hygge : Danish Secrets to Happy Living. New York, Ny, William Morrow, An Imprint Of Harpercollins Publishers, 2017

I know the strength of a Woman
because I have sat with Her.
She told me of the terrors of her childhood
The screaming and the shouting,
The silent tears.
I sat with her.
She recalled the day her baby brother died
at the hands of violence,
And I sat with her.
She told me about her barren womb,
Her desires that will never be fulfilled.
I sat with her.
She told me about her fears
That she'll fail as a mother.
I sat with her.
She told me about how she hit the floor
When her husband was diagnosed,
When her father died,
When she got news that ripped her open.
She told me about her persecution
for her actions marked with despair;
about her nights crying in the closet.
When no one sat with her.
She told me about how she held his clothes,
buttoned his dress shirts one by one,
she boxed them up.
Knowing that was the last of him.
And I sat with her.
I know the Strength of Woman.
because I sat with You.

i sat with her

originally published in
MM Publication 00
5Two Press

ACKNOWLEDGEMENTS
thank you for sitting with me.

My Husband, **Aaron Rud**, for honoring and understanding the Wheel of the Woman enough to make space for this book to be born.

My publisher and friend, **Sharissa Bradley**, for not taking no for an answer, for pulling this book out of me.

My parents, **Bob and Carole Spears**, for praising and loving a spirit that was developing differently.

My dear friends, *many of you.* I'm blessed with a circle of wild women. **Alicia Richardson**, **Tia Ellington**, **Adriane Alvarez** and **Ray Rantz**, for being consistent pillars in my adult life.

My childhood teachers, some of the women who celebrated me in my formative years. To name a few- **Linda Kilby**, **Pat Heckert**, **Moira Leppard**.

The women who have kept the lineages alive. Jane Hardwick Collings, Lisa Lister, Meggan Watterson, to name a few.

The Magdalenas. All of you out there. I see you. I love you.

Thank you.

about
MM

Kristen Rud is a visionary community leader. Her mission is to empower women towards a better quality of life by honoring the sacred rites of passage throughout their lives, using post-modern wellness as a guide.

She began her studies in early childhood education and intervention, where she grasped the importance of understanding psychophysiology for overall wellbeing and homeostasis. She continued on to complete a traditional midwifery program, and has assisted over 70 women through pregnancy and birth while building hundreds of feminine leaders up.

Kristen founded MM Women's Wellness, making waves in women's health and wellbeing. She is also the director of MM Publication and host of the annual women's event, Spiritual Summer Camp in Southern California.

While always a student, Kristen's leadership and commitment to women's wellness have made a valuable impact on communities across the country.

Kristen means Follower of Christ, with Egyptian roots, commonly used in Scandinavian cultures. I never resonated with my name. My mother chose it simply because she liked it. I always felt that it lacked depth or meaning. But now I know it was another way I was marked, to lead my lineage back to its roots. My love for Magdalene came before the knowledge of my bloodline connection (*brought to light in my acknowledgments at the beginning of this book*), mostly through the work of Meggan Watterson.

"I think we are finally ready for her teachings, for the other half of the story that began not with Christ's birth but with his resurrection. The story of a potential we all possess while we're human to be the bridge between heaven and earth. The story of a woman who was beloved to Christ not because she followed him, or worshiped him like an idol or a being far greater than she ever could be. But rather, because she followed his example and became the love that he was also.

And I would tell you that this love she became is what our world needs most desperately. It's a love that renders all things sacred, from the animals to the angels, from the poorest to the most powerful. It's a love that sees the inherent worth in all living things.

Mary Magdalene is the embodiment of a love that reaches where it never has before."
-*Meggan Watterson*

the wheel of the woman
is a calling back home.
it's a guide; not a rulebook.
it's a starting point to lead you
down the path towards your true nature;
to lead you back to love.
eve. woman. femme.
magdalene.
whatever you want to call her.

Xo, MM

Kristen Rud

the mm vision

We envision a world where women are valued for their unique perspectives and contributions, and where they have access to the resources and support they need to thrive. In this world, women are seen, heard, understood, and well

the mm mission

Our mission is to empower women towards a better quality of life through post-modern wellness practices that prioritize mental, physical, and emotional well-being. We believe seasonal living and community care are the foundational pieces of women's wellbeing.

www.mmwomenswellness.org
@mm.womenswellness

www.mmpublication.org
@mm.publication

@spiritualsummercamp